My Air Fryer Toaster Oven Daily Recipes

Quick And Easy Soup Recipes To Boost Your Metabolism

Eva Morris

TABLE OF CONTENT

this book has been derived from various sources. Please consult a licensed professional before attempting any techniques outlined in this book.

By reading this document, the reader agrees that under no circumstances is the author responsible for any losses, direct or indirect, which are incurred as a result of the use of information contained within this document, including, but not limited to, — errors, omissions, or inaccuracies.

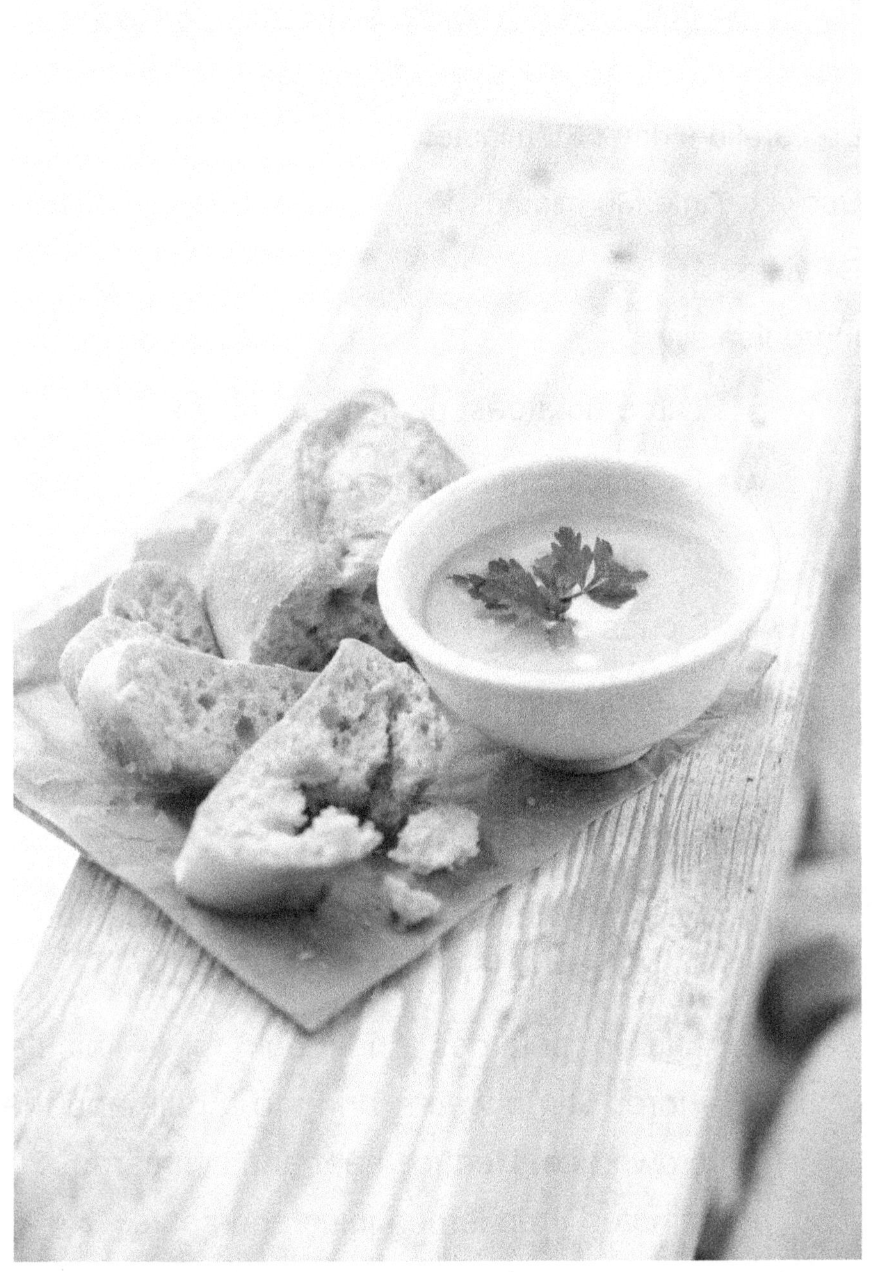

Leek, Brown Rice, And Potato Soup

Preparation Time: 35 minutes

Cooking Time: 30 minutes

Servings: 4

Ingredients:

- Three potatoes, peeled and diced
- Two leeks, finely chopped
- 1/4 cup brown rice
- 5 cups of water
- 3 tbsp. extra virgin olive oil
- Lemon juice, to taste.

Directions:

1. Heat olive oil in a deep soup pot and sauté leeks for 3-4 minutes.

2. Add in potatoes and cook for a minute more. Stir in water; bring to a boil, and the brown rice. Reduce heat and simmer for 30 minutes. Add lemon juice and serve.

Italian Mushroom And Kale Soup

Preparation Time: 35 minutes

Cooking Time: 20 minutes

Servings: 4

Ingredients:

- One onion, chopped
- One carrot, chopped
- One zucchini, peeled and diced
- One potato, peeled and diced
- Ten white mushrooms, chopped
- One bunch kale (10 oz.), stemmed and coarsely chopped
- 3 cups vegetable broth
- 4 tbsp. extra virgin olive oil
- salt and black pepper to taste

Directions:

1. Gently heat olive oil in a large soup pot.
2. Add in onions, carrot, and mushrooms and cook until vegetables are tender.

3. Stir in the zucchini, kale, and vegetable broth—season to taste with salt and pepper and simmer for 20 minutes.

Italian Chicken Soup

Preparation Time: 35 minutes

Cooking Time: 30 minutes

Servings: 4

Ingredients:

- Three chicken breasts, one carrot, chopped

- One small zucchini, peeled and chopped

- One celery stalk, chopped

- One small onion, chopped

- One bay leaf

- 5 cups water; 6-7 black olives, pitted and halved

- 1/2 tsp. Salt; 1 tsp. dried basil

- black pepper, fresh parsley, lemon juice, to serve

Directions:

1. Place chicken breasts, onion, carrot, celery, and bay leaf in a deep soup pot. Add in salt, black pepper, basil, and water.

2. Stir well and bring to a boil. Add zucchini and olives and reduce heat.

3. Simmer for 30 minutes. Remove chicken from the pot and set aside to cool. Serve with lemon juice and sprinkled with parsley.

Broccoli And Chicken Soup

Preparation Time: 35 minutes

Cooking Time: 30 minutes

Servings: 4

Ingredients:

- Four boneless chicken thighs, diced
- One small carrot, chopped
- One broccoli head, broken into florets
- One garlic clove, chopped
- One small onion, chopped
- 4 cups of water
- 3 tbsp. extra virgin olive oil
- 1/2 tsp. salt, black pepper, to taste

Directions:

1. In a deep soup pot, heat olive oil and gently sauté broccoli for 2-3 minutes, stirring occasionally. Add in onion, carrot, chicken, and cook, stirring, for 2-3 minutes.

2. Stir in salt, black pepper, and water. Bring to a boil.

3. Simmer for 30 minutes, then remove from heat and set aside to cool. In a blender or food processor, blend soup until completely smooth. Serve and enjoy!

Beef And Vegetable Soup

Preparation Time: 35 minutes

Cooking Time: 30 minutes

Servings: 4

Ingredients:

- Two slices bacon, chopped
- 1 lb. lean ground beef
- One carrot, chopped
- Two cloves garlic, finely chopped
- One small onion, chopped
- One celery stalk, chopped
- One bay leaf; 1 tsp. dried basil
- 1 cup canned tomatoes, diced and drained
- 4 cups beef broth
- 1/2 cup canned chickpeas
- ½ cup vermicelli Directions.

Directions:

1. In a large soup pot, cook bacon and ground beef until well done, breaking up the meat as it cooks. Drain off the fat and add in

onion, garlic, carrot, and celery.

2. Cook for 3-4 minutes until fragrant. Stir in the bay leaf, basil, tomatoes, and beef broth. Bring to a boil, then reduce heat and simmer for about 20 minutes.

3. Add the chickpeas and vermicelli. Cook, uncovered, for about 5 minutes more and serves.

Barley Beef Soup

Preparation Time: 35 minutes

Cooking Time: 30 minutes

Servings: 4

Ingredients:

- 12 oz. beef stew meat, cut into

- inch cubes one medium leek, chopped

- garlic cloves, chopped

- bay leaves

- can tomatoes (15 oz.), diced and drained

- 1/2 cup barley

- 1 cup of frozen mixed vegetables

- cups beef broth

- tbsp. extra virgin olive oil

- 1 tsp. paprika

Directions:

1. Heat oil in a large saucepan over medium-high heat. Sauté beef until well browned. Add in leeks and garlic and sauté until fragrant.

2. Add paprika, beef broth, and bay leaves; season with salt and pepper.

3. Cover and bring to a boil, then reduce heat and simmer for 60 minutes. Stir in frozen vegetables, tomatoes, and barley.

4. Return to boiling, reduce heat, and simmer, covered, about 15 minutes more or until meat and vegetables are tender. Discard bay leaves and serve.

Tuscan Bean Soup

Preparation Time: 35 minutes

Cooking Time: 30 minutes

Servings: 4

Ingredients:

- One onion, chopped
- One large carrot, chopped
- Two garlic cloves, minced
- 15 oz. can white beans, rinsed and drained
- 1 cup spinach leaves, trimmed and washed
- cups chicken broth
- 1 tbsp. paprika
- 1 tbsp. dried mint
- tbsp. extra virgin olive oil
- salt and black pepper, to taste

Directions

1. Heat the olive oil over medium heat and gently sauté the onion, garlic, and carrot.

2. Add in beans, broth, salt, and pepper and bring to a boil.

3. Reduce heat and cook for 10 minutes, or until the carrots are tender. Stir in spinach, and simmer for about 5 minutes, until spinach is wilted.

Meatball Soup

Preparation Time: 35 minutes

Cooking Time: 30 minutes

Servings: 4

Ingredients:

- 1 lb. lean ground beef
- ½ bunch of parsley, finely cut
- One egg, lightly whisked
- 1/2 onion, chopped
- Two garlic cloves, chopped
- 1/2 red bell pepper, chopped
- One tomato, diced
- two potatoes, diced
- four cups of water
- 4 tbsp. flour
- One cup vermicelli, broken into pieces
- 3 tbsp. extra virgin olive oil

- ½ tsp. black pepper

- 1 tsp. paprika

- 1 tsp. salt

Directions:

1. Place ground meat, egg, black pepper, and salt in a bowl. Combine well with hands and roll teaspoonful of the mixture into balls.

2. Place flour in a shallow bowl, roll each meatball in the flour and then set aside on a large plate.

3. Heat olive oil into a deep soup pot and gently sauté onion and garlic until transparent. Add water and bring to a boil. Stir in meatballs, carrot, pepper, tomato, and potatoes.

4. Reduce heat to low and simmer, uncovered, for 15 minutes. Add parsley and vermicelli and cook for five more minutes. Serve with a dollop of yogurt on top.

Mediterranean Chickpea Soup

Preparation Time: 35 minutes

Cooking Time: 20 minutes

Servings: 4

Ingredients:

- one can (15 oz.) chickpeas, drained
- one small onion, chopped
- One garlic cloves, minced
- One can (15 oz.) tomatoes, diced
- two cups vegetable broth
- one cup milk
- tbsp. extra virgin olive oil
- Two bay leaves
- 1/2 tsp. dried oregano

Directions:

1. Heat olive oil in a deep soup pot and sauté onion and garlic for 1-2 minutes.

2. Add in broth, chickpeas, tomatoes, bay leaves, and oregano.

3. Bring the soup to a boil, then reduce heat and simmer for 20 minutes.

4. Add in milk and cook for 1-2 minutes more. Set aside to cool, discard the bay leaves, and blend until smooth.

Italian Vegetable Soup

Preparation Time: 35 minutes

Cooking Time: 20 minutes

Servings: 4

Ingredients:

- 1/2 onion, chopped

- Two garlic cloves, chopped

- ¼ cabbage, chopped

- 3 cups water; 1 carrot, chopped

- Two celery stalks, chopped

- One cup canned tomatoes, diced, undrained

- One and a half cup green beans, trimmed and cut into

- 1/2-inch pieces

- 1/2 cup pasta, cooked

- 2-3 fresh basil leaves

- 2 tbsp. extra virgin olive oil

- black pepper and salt to taste

Directions:

1. Heat the olive oil in a large pot over medium-high heat.

2. Add the onion and cook until translucent, about 4 minutes.

3. Add in the garlic, carrot, and celery and cook for 5 minutes more.

4. Stir in the green beans, cabbage, tomatoes, basil, and water and bring to a boil.

5. Reduce heat and simmer uncovered for 15 minutes or until vegetables are tender. Stir in pasta, season with pepper and salt to taste, and serve.

Creamy Tomato And Roasted Pepper Soup

Preparation Time: 20 minutes

Cooking Time: 35 minutes

Servings: 4

Ingredients:

- one (12-ounce) jar roasted red peppers, drained and chopped
- one large onion, chopped
- two garlic cloves, minced
- Four medium tomatoes, chopped
- 4 cups vegetable broth
- 3 tbsp. extra virgin olive oil
- Two bay leaves

Directions:

1. Heat olive oil in a large saucepan over medium-high heat and sauté onion for 3-4 minutes, stirring. Add in garlic and sauté until just fragrant.

2. Stir in the red peppers, bay leaves, and tomatoes, and simmer for 10 minutes. Add broth, season with salt and pepper, and bring to the boil.

3. Reduce heat and simmer for 20 minutes. Set aside to cool slightly, remove the bay leaves and blend, in batches, until smooth.

Celery, Apple And Carrot Soup

Preparation Time: 20 minutes

Cooking Time: 15 minutes

Servings: 4

Ingredients:

- Two celery stalks, chopped
- 1/2 onion, chopped
- Two carrots, chopped
- 3-4 tbsp. extra virgin olive oil
- One large apple, chopped
- One garlic clove, minced
- 4 cups vegetable broth
- 1 tsp. paprika
- 1 tsp. grated ginger
- salt and black pepper, to taste

Directions:

1. Heat olive oil in a deep soup pot over medium-high heat.

2. Gently sauté onion, garlic, and carrots for 3 -4 minutes, stirring. Add in paprika, ginger, celery, apple, and broth.

3. Bring to the boil, and then reduce heat and simmer, covered, for 10 minutes. Blend the soup until smooth and return to pan. Cook over medium-high heat until heated through. Season with salt and pepper to taste and serve.

Bean And Pasta Soup

Preparation Time: 20 minutes

Cooking Time: 15 minutes

Servings: 4

Ingredients:

- One onion, chopped
- two large carrots, chopped
- two garlic cloves, minced
- One cup cooked orzo
- One 15 oz. canned can of white beans, rinsed and drained
- One 15 oz. can of tomatoes, diced and undrained
- One cup baby spinach leaves
- Three cups chicken broth
- 1 tbsp. Paprika; 1 tbsp. dried mint
- 3 tbsp. extra virgin olive oil
- salt and black pepper, to taste

Directions:

1. Heat the olive oil over medium heat and gently sauté the onion, garlic, and carrots.

2. Add in tomatoes, broth, salt, and pepper, and bring to a boil.

3. Reduce heat and cook for 5-10 minutes, or until the carrots are tender. Stir in orzo, beans, and spinach, and simmer until spinach is wilted.

Crispy Potato Wedges

Preparation Time: 10 minutes

Cooking Time: 15 minutes

Serve: 4

Ingredients:

- Two medium potatoes, cut into wedges
- 1/8 tsp. cayenne pepper
- 1/4 tsp. garlic powder
- 1/2 tsp. paprika
- 1 1/2 tbsp. olive oil
- 1/4 tsp. pepper
- 1 tsp. sea salt

Directions:

1. Soak potato wedges into the cold water for 30 minutes. Drain well and pat dry with a paper towel.

2. In a mixing bowl, toss potato wedges with remaining ingredients.

3. Insert wire rack in rack position 4. Select air fry, set temperature 400 F, timer for 15 minutes. Press start to preheat the oven.

4. Arrange potato wedges in the air fryer basket and cook for 15 minutes.

5. Serve and enjoy.

Nutrition:

Calories 120

Fat 5.4 g

Carbohydrates 17.1 g

Sugar 1.3 g

Protein 1.9 g

Cholesterol 0 mg

Thyme Parmesan Potatoes

Preparation Time: 10 minutes

Cooking Time: 45 minutes

Serve: 4

Ingredients:

- Five potatoes, cut into wedges
- 2 tbsp. lemon juice
- 1/3 cup olive oil
- Two garlic cloves, minced
- Two thyme sprigs
- 1/2 cup parmesan cheese, grated
- Pepper
- Salt

Directions:

1. Spray a 9*13-inch baking dish with cooking spray and set aside.

2. Insert wire rack in rack position 4. Select bake, set temperature 325 F, timer for 45 minutes. Press start to preheat the oven.

3. Add potato wedges into the baking dish.

4. Mix lemon juice, oil, garlic, thyme, cheese, pepper, and salt and pour over potatoes and toss well.

5. Bake for 45 minutes.

6. Serve and enjoy.

Nutrition:

Calories 374

Fat 19.7 g

Carbohydrates 44.3 g

Sugar 3.3 g

Protein 8.5 g

Cholesterol 8 mg

Easy Buffalo Chicken Dip

Preparation Time: 10 minutes

Cooking Time: 25 minutes

Serve: 8

Ingredients:

- Two chicken breasts, skinless, boneless, cooked and shredded
- 1 cup Monterey jack cheese, shredded
- 1 cup cheddar cheese, shredded
- 1/4 cup blue cheese, crumbled
- 1/2 cup ranch dressing
- 1/2 cup buffalo wing sauce
- 8 oz. cream cheese, softened

Directions:

1. Spray a 1.5-quart casserole dish with cooking spray and set aside.

2. Insert wire rack in rack position 4. Select bake, set temperature 350 F, timer for 25 minutes. Press start to preheat the oven.

3. Add cream cheese into the casserole dish and top with shredded chicken, ranch dressing, and buffalo sauce.

4. Sprinkle cheddar cheese, Monterey jack cheese, and blue cheese on top of chicken mixture.

5. Bake for 25 minutes.

6. Serve and enjoy.

Nutrition):

Calories 298

Fat 22.8 g

Carbohydrates 2 g

Sugar 0.6 g

Protein 20.8 g

Cholesterol 94 mg

Perfect Goat Cheese Dip

Preparation Time: 10 minutes

Cooking Time: 20 minutes

Serve: 8

Ingredients:

- 12 oz. goat cheese
- 2 tsp. rosemary, chopped
- 1 tsp. red pepper flakes
- Four garlic cloves, minced
- 2 tbsp. olive oil
- 1/2 cup parmesan cheese, shredded
- 4 oz. cream cheese
- 1/2 tsp. salt

Directions:

1. Spray a baking dish with cooking spray and set aside.

2. Insert wire rack in rack position 4. Select bake, set temperature 390 F, timer for 20 minutes. Press start to preheat the oven.

3. Add all ingredients into the mixing bowl and mix until well combined. Pour mixture into the baking dish and bake for 20 minutes.

4. Serve and enjoy.

Nutrition:

Calories 294

Fat 24.9 g

Carbohydrates 2.3 g

Sugar 1 g

Protein 16 g

Cholesterol 64 mg

Easy Taco Dip

Preparation Time: 10 minutes

Cooking Time: 25 minutes

Serve: 2

Ingredients:

- 1/4 cup salsa

- 2 tbsp. red pepper, chopped

- 2 tbsp. onion, chopped

- 1 cup cheddar cheese, shredded

- 1/2 cup sour cream

- 1/2 cup miracle whip

- 1 oz. taco seasoning

Directions:

1. Spray a baking dish with cooking spray and set aside.

2. Insert wire rack in rack position 4. Select bake, set temperature 350 F, timer for 25 minutes. Press start to preheat the oven.

3. In a bowl, mix all ingredients and pour into the baking dish and bake for 25 minutes.

4. Serve and enjoy.

Nutrition:

Calories 661

Fat 52.5 g

Carbohydrates 31.4 g

Sugar 11.6 g

Protein 19.9 g

Cholesterol 105 mg

Spicy Mexican Cheese Dip

Preparation Time: 10 minutes

Cooking Time: 30 minutes

Serve: 10

Ingredients:

- 16 oz. cream cheese softened

- 1/2 cup hot salsa

- 3 cups cheddar cheese, shredded

- 1 cup sour cream

Directions:

1. Spray an 8*8-inch baking dish with cooking spray and set aside.

2. Insert wire rack in rack position 4. Select bake, set temperature 350 F, timer for 25 minutes. Press start to preheat the oven.

3. In a mixing bowl, mix all ingredients until well combined and pour into the baking dish and bake for 30 minutes.

4. Serve and enjoy.

Nutrition:

Calories 348

Fat 31.9 g

Carbohydrates 3.4 g

Sugar 0.7 g

Protein 12.8 g

Cholesterol 96 mg

Cheese Garlic Dip

Preparation Time: 10 minutes

Cooking Time: 8 minutes

Serve: 6

Ingredients:

- 13 oz. brie cheese, remove the rind and cubed
- 1 tbsp. dried thyme
- 2 tsp. rosemary, chopped
- Three garlic cloves, chopped
- Pepper
- Salt

Directions:

1. Spray a baking dish with cooking spray and set aside.

2. Insert wire rack in rack position 4. Select bake, set temperature 375 F, timer for 8 minutes. Press start to preheat the oven.

3. Add all ingredients into the mixing bowl and mix well. Pour mixture into the baking

dish and bake for 8 minutes.

4. Serve and enjoy.

Nutrition:

Calories 210

Fat 17.1 g

Carbohydrates 1.3 g

Sugar 0.3 g

Protein 12.9 g

Cholesterol 61 mg

Cheesy Crab Dip

Preparation Time: 10 minutes

Cooking Time: 15 minutes

Serve: 4

Ingredients:

- 8 oz. crab meat
- 1/4 tsp. paprika
- 1/2 tsp. garlic powder
- 1/4 cup onion, chopped
- 1 1/2 tsp. garlic, minced
- 1 cup cheddar cheese, shredded
- 1/2 cup sour cream
- 1/4 cup mayonnaise
- 8 oz. cream cheese, softened
- Pepper
- Salt

Directions:

1. Spray a baking dish with cooking spray and set aside.

2. Insert wire rack in rack position 4. Select bake, set temperature 390 F, timer for 15 minutes. Press start to preheat the oven.

3. Add all ingredients into the bowl and mix until well combined. Pour mixture into the baking dish and bake for 15 minutes.

4. Serve and enjoy.

Nutrition:

Calories 487

Fat 41.1 g

Carbohydrates 9 g

Sugar 1.7 g

Protein 19.7 g

Cholesterol 139 mg

Broccoli Nuggets

Preparation Time: 10 minutes

Cooking Time: 20 minutes

Serve: 4

Ingredients:

- 1/4 cup almond flour
- 2 cups broccoli florets, cooked until soften
- 1 cup cheddar cheese, shredded
- Two egg whites
- 1/8 tsp. salt

Directions:

1. Line baking sheet with parchment paper and set aside.

2. Insert wire rack in rack position 6. Select bake, set temperature 350 F, timer for 20 minutes. Press start to preheat the oven.

3. Add cooked broccoli to the bowl, and using a masher, mash broccoli into small pieces.

4. Add remaining ingredients to the bowl and mix until well combined.

5. Drop 20 scoops of broccoli mixture onto the prepared baking sheet and press into a nugget shape.

6. Bake for 20 minutes.

7. Serve and enjoy.

Nutrition:

Calories 180

Fat 12.9 g

Carbohydrates 5 g

Sugar 1 g

Protein 11.6 g

Cholesterol 30 mg

Stuffed Jalapenos

Preparation Time: 10 minutes

Cooking Time: 25 minutes

Serve: 12

Ingredients:

- Six jalapenos halved

- 1/4 cup green onion, sliced

- 1/4 cup Monterey jack cheese, shredded

- 1/4 tsp. dried basil

- 1/2 cup chicken, cooked and shredded

- 1/4 tsp. garlic powder

- 4 oz. cream cheese

- 1/4 tsp. dried oregano

- 1/4 tsp. salt

Directions:

1. Line baking sheet with parchment paper and set aside.

2. Insert wire rack in rack position 6. Select bake, set temperature 390 F, timer for 25 minutes. Press start to preheat the oven.

3. Mix all ingredients in a bowl except jalapenos.

4. Spoon one tablespoon mixture into each jalapeno half and place it on a baking sheet.

5. Bake for 25 minutes.

6. Serve and enjoy.

Nutrition:

Calories 54

Fat 4.2 g

Carbohydrates 0.9 g

Sugar 0.3 g

Protein 3.1 g

Cholesterol 17 mg

Broccoli Fritters

Preparation Time: 10 minutes

Cooking Time: 30 minutes

Serve: 4

Ingredients:

- 3 cups broccoli florets, steam & chopped
- 2 cups cheddar cheese, shredded
- 1/4 cup almond flour
- Two eggs, lightly beaten
- Two garlic cloves, minced
- **Pepper**
- **Salt**

Directions:

1. Line baking sheet with parchment paper and set aside.

2. Insert wire rack in rack position 6. Select bake, set temperature 375 F, timer for 15 minutes. Press start to preheat the oven.

3. Add all ingredients into the large bowl and mix until well combined.

4. Make patties from broccoli mixture and place on a baking sheet, and bake for 15 minutes.

5. Turn patties and bake for 15 minutes more.

6. Serve and enjoy.

Nutrition:

Calories 327

Fat 24.5 g

Carbohydrates 7.4 g

Sugar 2.6 g

Protein 20.4 g

Cholesterol 141 mg

Ranch Potatoes

Preparation Time: 10 minutes

Cooking Time: 20 minutes

Serve: 2

Ingredients:

- 1/2 lb. baby potatoes, wash and cut in half
- 1/2 tbsp. olive oil
- 1/4 tsp. dill
- 1/4 tsp. chives
- 1/4 tsp. paprika
- 1/4 tsp. onion powder
- 1/4 tsp. garlic powder
- 1/4 tsp. parsley
- **Salt**

Directions:

1. Insert wire rack in rack position 4. Select air fry, set temperature 400 F, timer for 10 minutes. Press start to preheat the oven.

2. Add all ingredients into the mixing bowl and toss well.

3. Spread potatoes on an air fryer basket and air fry for 20 minutes.

4. Serve and enjoy.

Nutrition:

Calories 99

Fat 3.7 g

Carbohydrates 14.8 g

Sugar 0.2 g

Protein 3.1 g

Cholesterol 0 mg

Potato Nuggets

Preparation Time: 10 minutes

Cooking Time: 42 minutes

Serve: 4

Ingredients:

- 2 cups potatoes, chopped
- One garlic clove, minced
- 1 tsp. olive oil
- 2 tbsp. almond milk
- 4 cups kale, chopped
- **Pepper**
- **Salt**

Directions:

1. Insert wire rack in rack position 4. Select air fry, set temperature 390 F, timer for 12 minutes. Press start to preheat the oven.

2. Add potatoes in boiling water and cook for 30 minutes or until tender. Drain well.

3. Heat oil in a pan over medium-high heat.

4. Add garlic and sauté for 30 seconds. Add kale and sauté for 2 minutes.

5. Transfer sautéed garlic and kale in a large bowl. Add potatoes, almond milk, pepper, salt, and mash potato using a fork and stir to combine.

6. Make small nuggets from potato mixture and place on an air fryer basket, and air fry for 12 minutes.

7. Serve and enjoy.

Nutrition:

Calories 113

Fat 3 g

Carbohydrates 19.5 g

Sugar 1.1 g

Protein 3.5 g

Cholesterol 0 mg

Tasty Zucchini Patties

Preparation Time: 10 minutes

Cooking Time: 25 minutes

Serve: 6

Ingredients:

- 1 cup zucchini, shredded and squeeze out all liquid
- 2 tbsp. onion, minced
- One egg, lightly beaten
- 1/4 tsp. red pepper flakes
- 1/4 cup parmesan cheese, grated
- 1/2 tbsp. Dijon mustard
- 1/2 tbsp. mayonnaise
- 1/2 cup breadcrumbs
- **Pepper**
- **Salt**

Directions:

1. Insert wire rack in rack position 4. Select air fry, set temperature 400 F, timer for 25

minutes. Press start to preheat the oven.

2. Add all ingredients into the bowl and mix until well combined.

3. Make small patties from the zucchini mixture, place it on an air fryer basket, and air fry for 25 minutes.

4. Serve and enjoy.

Nutrition:

Calories 68

Fat 2.5 g

Carbohydrates 8 g

Sugar 1.2 g

Protein 3.7 g

Cholesterol 30 mg

Roasted Broccoli Cauliflower

Preparation Time: 5 minutes

Cooking Time: 15 minutes

Serve: 12

Ingredients:

- 4 cups broccoli florets
- 2/3 cup parmesan cheese, grated and divided
- 4 cups cauliflower florets
- Six garlic cloves, minced
- 1/3 cup olive oil
- Pepper
- Salt

Directions:

1. Preheat the oven to 400 F.
2. Spray a baking dish with cooking spray and set aside.
3. Add cauliflower, broccoli, half cheese, garlic, and olive oil in a bowl and toss well

—season with pepper and salt.

4. Arrange broccoli and cauliflower mixture on a prepared baking dish.

5. Select bake mode and set the Omni to 400 F for 15 minutes once the oven beeps, place the baking dish into the oven.

6. Just before serving, add remaining cheese and toss well.

7. Serve and enjoy.

Nutritional Value (Amount per Serving):

Calories 86

Fat 6.9 g

Carbohydrates 4.5 g

Sugar 1.3 g

Protein 3.4 g

Cholesterol 4 mg

Baked Egg Tomato

Preparation Time: 5 minutes

Cooking Time: 30 minutes

Serve: 2

Ingredients:

- 2 eggs

    - 1 tsp. fresh parsley

    - 2 large fresh tomatoes

- Pepper

- Salt

Directions:

1. Cut the top of the tomato and spoon out the tomato innards.

2. Break the egg in each tomato. Place tomatoes on the cooking pan.

3. Select bake mode and set the omni to 350 F for 30 minutes once the oven beeps, place the cooking pan into the oven.

4. Season with pepper, and salt.

5. Garnish with parsley and serve.

Nutritional Value (Amount per Serving):

Calories 96

Fat 4.7 g

Carbohydrates 7.5 g

Sugar 5.1 g

Protein 7.2 g

Cholesterol 164 mg

Veggie Tots

Preparation Time: 10 minutes

Cooking Time: 10 minutes

Serve: 2

Ingredients:

- 1 egg

    - 1 carrot, grated & squeeze out the liquid

    - 1/4 cup breadcrumbs

    - 1 zucchini, grated & squeeze out the liquid

    - 1/4 cup parmesan cheese, grated

- Pepper

- Salt

Directions:

1. Spray air fryer basket with cooking spray.

2. Add all ingredients into the bowl and mix until well combined.

3. Make tots from mixture and place into the air fryer basket.

4. Place air fryer basket into the oven and select air fry mode set omni to the 400 F for 15 minutes.

5. Serve and enjoy.

Nutrition:

Calories 153

Fat 5.8 g

Carbohydrates 16.7 g

Sugar 4.2 g

Protein 10 g

Cholesterol 91 mg

Tasty Potato Fries

Preparation Time: 10 minutes

Cooking Time: 20 minutes

Serve: 2

Ingredients:

- 1 lb potatoes, wash, peel and cut into fries shape

- 1/4 tsp chili powder

- 1/2 tbsp olive oil

- 1/4 tsp smoked paprika

- Salt

Directions:

1. Spray air fryer basket with cooking spray.

2. Add potato fries in a large bowl and drizzle with olive oil. Season with paprika, chili powder, and salt.

3. Add potato fries into the air fryer basket.

4. Place air fryer basket into the oven and select air fry mode set omni to the 370 F for 20 minutes. Stir twice.

5. Serve and enjoy.

Nutrition:

Calories 188

Fat 3.8 g

Carbohydrates 36 g

Sugar 2.7 g

Protein 3.9 g

Cholesterol 0 mg

Baby Potatoes

Preparation Time: 10 minutes

Cooking Time: 20 minutes

Serve: 2

Ingredients:

- 12 oz. baby potatoes
- 1/4 tsp. cumin
- 1/4 tsp. paprika
- 1/4 tsp. chili powder
- 1/2 tbsp. olive oil
- 1/4 tsp. garlic salt
- 1/4 tsp. pepper
- 1/2 tsp. kosher salt

Directions:

1. Add all ingredients into a zip-lock bag and shake well.

2. Transfer potatoes into the air fryer basket.

3. Place air fryer basket into the oven and select air fry mode set omni to the 370 F

for 20 minutes. Stir twice.

4. Serve and enjoy.

Nutrition:

Calories 133

Fat 3.8 g

Carbohydrates 22 g

Sugar 0.2 g

Protein 4.6 g

Cholesterol 0 mg

Parmesan Hassel Back Potatoes

Preparation Time: 10 minutes

Cooking Time: 40 minutes

Serve: 2

Ingredients:

- 2 potatoes make the thin slices

- 2tbsps. butter, melted

- tbsps. mushrooms, sliced

- 4 tbsps. parmesan cheese, grated

- Pepper

- Salt

Directions:

1. Spray the cooking pan with cooking spray and set aside.

2. Slide mushroom slices into each slit.

3. Place potatoes on cooking pan and brush with half-melted butter.

4. Place cooking pan into the oven and select air fry mode set omni to the 350 F for 20 minutes.

5. Turn potatoes to the other side and brush with remaining butter and air fry for 20 minutes more.

6. Sprinkle with parmesan cheese and serve.

Nutrition:

Calories 345

Fat 18 g

Carbohydrates 34.8 g

Sugar 2.6 g

Protein 13.4 g

Cholesterol 51 mg

Masala Gillette

Preparation Time: 10 minutes

Cooking Time: 35 minutes

Serving: 4

INGREDIENTS

- 2 - tbsp. garam masala

- 2 - medium potatoes boiled and mashed

- 1 ½ - cup coarsely crushed peanuts

- 3 - tsp. ginger finely chopped

- 1 to 2 - tbsp. fresh coriander leaves

- 2 or 3 - green chilies finely chopped

- 1 ½ - tbsp. lemon juice

- Salt and pepper to taste

Directions:

1. Blend the ingredients in a bowl.

2. Form this blend into round, flat galettes.

3. Wet the galettes with a small amount of water. Coat each galette with crushed peanuts.

4. Preheat the Air Fryer to 160 F for 5 minutes.

5. Place the galettes in the fry bin and let them cook for an additional 25 minutes.

6. Continue turning them over to cook uniformly.

7. Serve with mint chutney or ketchup.

Potato Samosa

Preparation Time: 10 minutes

Cooking Time: 30minutes

Serving: 4

INGREDIENTS

For wrappers:

- 2 - tbsp. unsalted butter
- 1 ½ - cup all-purpose flour
- A pinch of salt
- Water

For filling:

- 2 to 3 - large potatoes
- ¼ - cup boiled peas
- 1 - tsp. powdered ginger
- 1 or 2 - green chilies
- ½ - tsp. cumin
- 1 - tsp. coarsely crushed coriander
- 1 - dry red chili

- A small amount of salt

- ½ - tsp. mango powder

- ½ - tsp. Red chili powder.

- 1 to 2 - tbsp. Coriander.

Directions:

1. Blend the wrapper ingredients. Let it sit while making the filling.

2. Cook the ingredients in a skillet and blend them well to make a thick paste.

3. Form the paste into balls. Cut them in half and insert the filling.

4. Preheat the Air Fryer to 300 F. Place the samosas in the fry receptacle.

5. Cook for 20-25 minutes. Flip halfway through for uniform cooking.

6. Serve hot with tamarind or mint chutney.

Vegetable Kebab

Preparation Time: 10 minutes

Cooking Time: 25 minutes

Serving: 4

INGREDIENTS

- 2 cups of mixed vegetables
- Three onions chopped
- Five green chilies-roughly chopped
- 1 ½ tbsp. ginger paste
- 1 ½ tsp. garlic paste
- 1 ½ tsp. salt
- 3 tsp. lemon juice
- 2 tsp. garam masala
- 4 tbsp. chopped coriander
- 3 tbsp. cream
- 3 tbsp. chopped capsicum
- Three eggs
- 2 ½ tbsp. white sesame seeds

Directions:

1. Mix the ingredients except for the egg and form a smooth paste.

2. Coat the vegetables in the paste. Beat in the eggs and add salt to season.

3. Dip the vegetables in the egg mix and coat well with sesame seed.

4. Place the vegetables on skewers.

5. Preheat the Air fryer to 160 F. Cook for 25 minutes.

6. Turn the sticks over halfway through to cook uniformly.

Sago Galette

Preparation Time: 10 minutes

Cooking Time: 35 minutes

Serving: 4

INGREDIENTS

- 2 cup sago, soaked
- 1 ½ cup coarsely crushed peanuts
- 3 tsp. ginger finely chopped
- 1-2 tbsp. fresh coriander leaves
- 2 or 3 green chilies finely chopped
- 1 ½ tbsp. lemon juice
- Salt and pepper to taste

Directions:

1. Blend the ingredients in a bowl.

2. Form this blend into round, flat galettes.

3. Wet the galettes with a small amount of water. Coat each galette with crushed

peanuts.

4. Preheat the Air Fryer to 160 F for 5 minutes. Place the galettes in the fry bin and let them cook for an additional 25 minutes. Continue turning them over to cook uniformly.

5. Serve with mint chutney or ketchup.

Stuffed Capsicum Baskets

Preparation Time: 10 minutes

Cooking Time: 35 minutes

Serving: 4

INGREDIENTS

For baskets:

- 3-4 long capsicum
- ½ tsp. Salt
- ½ tsp. pepper powder

For filling:

- One medium onion
- One green chili
- 2 or 3 large potatoes
- 1 ½ tbsp. chopped coriander leaves
- 1 tsp. fenugreek
- 1 tsp. dried mango powder
- 1 tsp. cumin powder
- Salt and pepper

For topping:

- 3 tbsp. grated cheese
- 1 tsp. Red chili flakes
- ½ tsp. Oregano
- ½ tsp. Basil
- ½ tsp. parsley

Directions:

1. Mix all of the filling ingredients in a bowl.

2. Remove the stem, seeds, and top of the capsicum.

3. Sprinkle some salt and pepper inside the capsicums. Set aside.

4. Place the filling inside the peppers, leaving a little space at the top.

5. Mix topping spices and sprinkle ground cheese and seasoning on top.

6. Preheat the Air Fryer to 140 F for 5 minutes.

7. Put the capsicums in the fry case and cook for 20 minutes.

Macaroni Samosa

Preparation Time: 10 minutes

Cooking Time: 25 minutes

Serving: 4

INGREDIENTS

For wrappers:

- cup all-purpose flour
- 2- tbsp. unsalted butter
- A pinch of salt to taste
- Take the amount of water sufficient

For filling:

- 3- cups boiled macaroni
- 2- onion
- 2- capsicum
- 2- Carrots
- 2- Cabbage

- 2- tbsp. soy sauce

- 2- tsp. vinegar

- 2- tbsp. ginger

- 2- tbsp. garlic

- 2- tbsp. green chilies

- 2- tbsp. ginger-garlic paste

- Some salt and pepper

- 2- tbsp. olive oil

Directions:

1. Blend the wrapper ingredients until smooth. Set aside while making the filling.

2. Boil the filling ingredients and blend them to make a thick paste.

3. Form the batter into balls. Cut them in half and insert the filling.

4. Preheat the Air Fryer to 300 F. Place the samosas in the fry holder and cook for 20 to 25 minutes

5. Around the midpoint, turn the samosas over for uniform cooking.

6. Serve hot with tamarind or mint chutney.

Burritos

Preparation Time: 10 minutes

Cooking Time: 35 minutes

Serving: 4

INGREDIENTS

Refried beans:

- ½ cup red kidney beans
- ½ small onion
- 1 tbsp. olive oil
- 2 tbsp. Tomato puree
- ¼ tsp. red chili powder
- 1 tsp. of salt
- 4-5 flour tortillas

Vegetable Filling:

- 1 tbsp. Olive oil

- One medium onion

- Three flakes garlic crushed

- ½ cup French beans

- 1 cup cottage cheese

- ½ cup shredded cabbage

- 1 tbsp. coriander

- 1 tbsp. vinegar

- 1 tsp. white wine

- A pinch of salt

- ½ tsp. red chili flakes

- 1 tsp. freshly ground peppercorns

- ½ cup pickled Jalapeño s

- Two carrots

Salad:

- 1-2 lettuce leaves shredded.

- 1 or 2 spring onions

- One green chili

- 1 cup of cheddar

Directions:

1. Cook the beans with the onion and garlic and mash them.

2. For the filling, sauté the ingredients in a pan.

3. Toss the salad ingredients together.

4. Lay the tortilla on a flat surface and place a layer of sauce and filling inside.

5. Wrap the tortilla to create a burrito.

6. Preheat the Air Fryer to 200 F. Open the fry case and place the burritos inside.

7. Cook for 15 minutes. Flip the burritos halfway through.

Cheese And Bean Enchiladas

Preparation Time: 10 minutes

Cooking Time: 25 minutes

Serving: 4

INGREDIENTS

- Flour tortillas

Red sauce:

- 4 tbsp. of olive oil
- 1 ½ tsp. of garlic
- 1 ½ cups of readymade tomato puree
- Three medium tomatoes
- 1 tsp. of sugar
- A pinch of salt
- A few red chili flakes to sprinkle
- 1 tsp. of oregano

Filling:

- 2 tbsp. oil

- 2 tsp. chopped garlic

- Two onions

- Two capsicums

- 2 cups of readymade baked beans

- A few drops of Tabasco sauce

- 1 cup cottage cheese

- 1 cup grated cheddar

- A pinch of salt

- 1 tsp. Oregano

- ½ tsp. pepper

- 1 ½ tsp. red chili flakes

- 1 tbsp. of finely chopped Jalapeño s

Directions:

1. In a skillet, heat 2 tbsp. Of oil. Add garlic and the rest of the sauce ingredients.

2. Cook until the sauce reduces and ends up being thick.

3. For the filling, warm one tbsp. Of oil in another skillet.

4. Add onions and garlic and cook till the onions are caramelized.

5. Add the filling ingredients. Remove from heat and sprinkle Cheddar over the sauce.

6. Take a tortilla and spread a portion of the sauce on it. Roll up the tortilla cautiously and then repeat for each.

7. Line a baking pan with aluminum foil. Preheat the Air Fryer to 160° C and cook for 15 minutes.

8. Turn the tortillas over in the middle to cook uniformly.

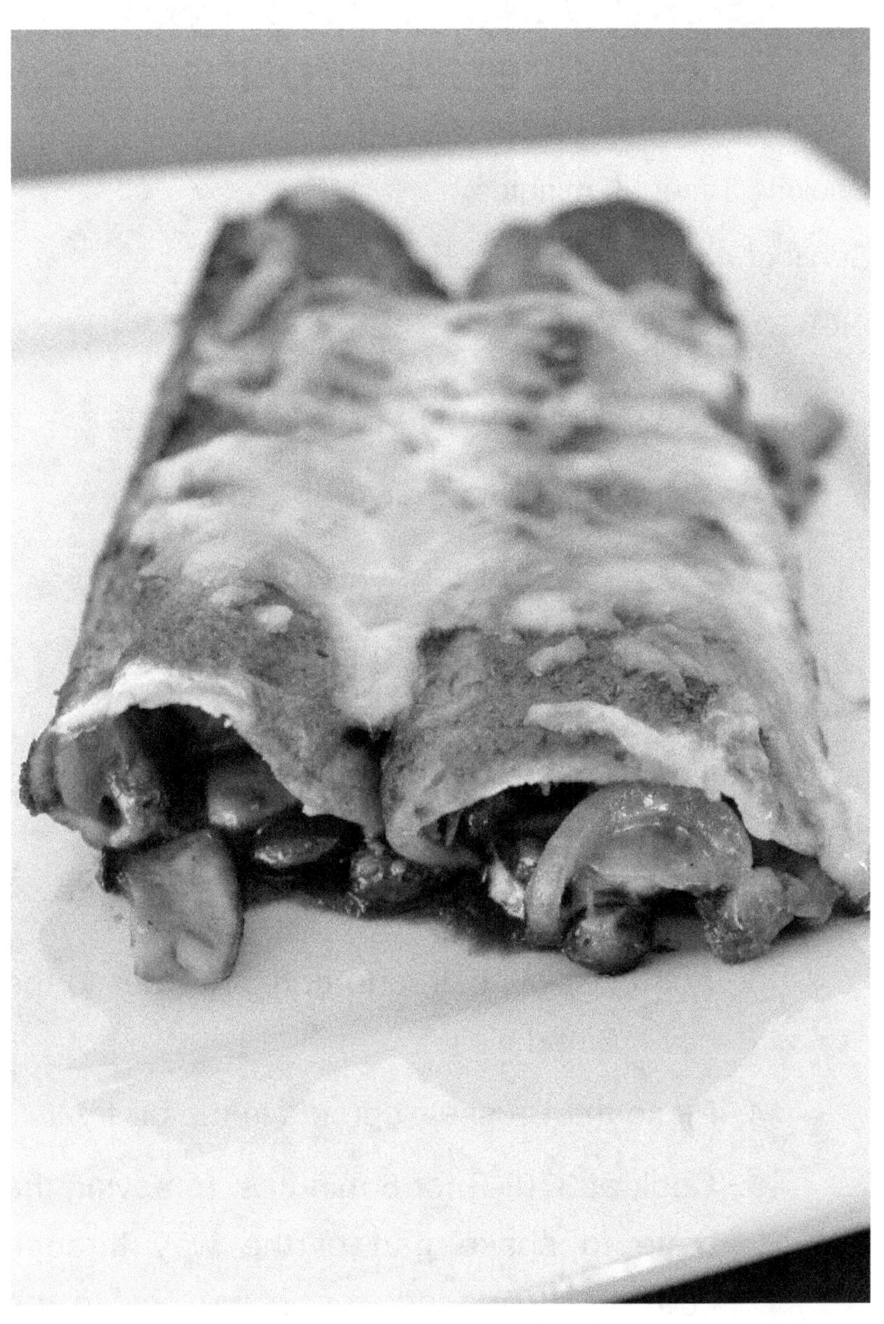

Easy Vegan Air Fryer Brussels Sprouts

Preparation Time: 10 minutes

Cooking Time: 20 minutes

Serving: 4

INGREDIENTS

- 1-pound Brussels Sprouts
- 2 tsp. olive oil
- 1/4 tsp. salt
- 1/4 tsp. garlic powder

Directions:

1. Prepare Brussels sprouts by cutting off the stem and any dark-colored leaves.

2. Place clean Brussels sprouts in a bowl.

3. Add olive oil, salt, and garlic powder to the bowl. Blend well.

4. Place the Brussels sprouts in the air fryer.

5. Cook at 370° F for 6 minutes, removing the crate to shake part of the way through cooking. If needed, return the box to the

air fryer and cook for 2-4 additional minutes.

Vegetable Momos

Preparation Time: 10 minutes

Cooking Time: 25 minutes

Serving: 4

INGREDIENTS

For dough:

- 1 ½ cup all-purpose flour
- ½ tsp. salt or to taste
- 5 tbsp. water

For filling:

- 2 cup carrots, grated
- 2 cup cabbage, grated
- 2 tbsp. oil
- 2 tsp. ginger-garlic paste
- 2 tsp. soy sauce
- 2 tsp. vinegar

Directions:

1. Mix the dough ingredients, cover it with plastic wrap, and set aside.

2. Sauté the filling ingredients.

3. Fold the dough and cut it into squares.
    Drop a spoonful of the filling in the center.
    Wrap the dough around the filling and
    press edges together.

4. Preheat the Air Fryer to 200° F and cook
    for 20 minutes. Serve with chili or
    ketchup.

Cornflakes French Toast

Preparation Time: 10 minutes

Cooking Time: 25 minutes

Serving: 4

INGREDIENTS

- Bread slices (brown or white)
- One egg white for every two slices
- 1 tsp. sugar for every two slices
- Crushed cornflakes

Directions:

1. Cut bread slices in half.

2. In a bowl, whisk the egg whites and sugar.

3. Dip the bread into this blend and then spread them with crushed cornflakes.

4. Preheat the Air Fryer to 180° C and cook for 20 minutes.

5. Flip the toast halfway through to cook uniformly.

6. Serve with chocolate sauce.

12. Smoky Air Fryer Chickpeas

INGREDIENTS

- 1 15 oz. can chickpeas

- 1 tsp. sunflower oil

- 2 tsp. Lemon juice and 3/4 tsp. smoked paprika

- 1/2 tsp. ground cumin

- 1/2 tsp. garlic

- 1/4 tsp. onion

- 1/2 tsp. sea salt

Directions:

1. Set your Air Fryer to 390 ° F.

2. Put the rinsed chickpeas in the bin and fry for 12 minutes.

3. Shake bin once at the halfway point.

4. In a medium bowl, mix the oil, lemon, and seasonings.

5. Add the seared chickpeas to the bowl of seasonings.

6. Put the prepared chickpeas back in your air fryer basket and set to 360 ° F. Fry for 2-3 minutes more.

Mint Galette

Preparation Time: 10 minutes

Cooking Time: 30 minutes

Serving: 4

INGREDIENTS

- 2 cups mint leaves, finely sliced
- Two medium potatoes, boiled and mashed
- 1 ½ cup coarsely crushed peanuts
- 3 tsp. ginger, finely chopped
- 1-2 tbsp. fresh coriander leaves
- 2 or 3 green chilies, finely chopped
- 1 ½ tbsp. lemon juice
- Salt and pepper to taste

Directions:

1. Blend the cut mint leaves in with the rest of the ingredients in a bowl.

2. Shape into galettes.

3. Wet the galettes with water. Coat each galette with crushed peanuts.

4. Preheat the Air Fryer to 160 F and cook for 25 minutes.

5. Shake occasionally to cook uniformly. Serve with mint chutney or ketchup.

Air Fryer Fruit Crumble

Preparation Time: 10 minutes

Cooking Time: 25 minutes

Serving: 4

INGREDIENTS

- One medium apple, finely diced

- 1/2 cup frozen blueberries or strawberries

- 1 1/4 cup brown rice flour

- 2 tsp. sugar

- 1/2 tsp. ground cinnamon

- 2 tbsp. non-dairy butter

Directions:

1. Preheat air fryer to 350°F for 5 minutes.

2. Place the apple and solidified berries in an air fryer-safe heating skillet or ramekin.

3. In a bowl, mix part of the flour, sugar, cinnamon, and butter.

4. Spoon the flour combo over the fruit.

5. Bake at 350° F for 15 minutes.

Palak Galette

Preparation Time: 10 minutes

Cooking Time: 40 minutes

Serving: 4

INGREDIENTS

- 2 tbsp. garam masala

- 2 cups palak leaves

- 1 ½ cup coarsely crushed peanuts

- 3 tsp. ginger finely chopped

- 1-2 tbsp. fresh coriander leaves

- 2 or 3 green chilies finely chopped

- 1 ½ tbsp. lemon juice

- Salt and pepper to taste

Directions:

1. Blend the ingredients in a bowl.

2. Form this blend into round, flat galettes.

3. Wet the galettes with a small amount of water. Coat each galette with crushed peanuts.

4. Preheat the Air Fryer to 160 F for 5 minutes.

5. Place the galettes in the fry bin and let them cook for an additional 25 minutes.

6. Continue turning them over to cook uniformly.

Serve with mint chutney or ketchup

Creamy Chicken Soup

Preparation Time: 35 minutes

Cooking Time: 30 minutes

Servings: 4

Ingredients:

- Four chicken breasts
- One carrot, chopped
- 1 cup zucchini, peeled and chopped
- 2 cups cauliflower, broken into florets
- One celery rib Chopped
- One small onion, chopped
- 5 cups of water
- 1/2 tsp. black pepper

Directions:

1. Place chicken breasts, onion, carrot, celery, cauliflower, and zucchini in a deep soup pot. Add in salt, black pepper, and 5 cups of water.

2. Stir and bring to a boil. Simmer for 30 minutes, then remove chicken from the pot and let it cool slightly. Blend the soup until completely smooth.

3. Shred or dice the chicken meat, return it to the pot, stir and serve.

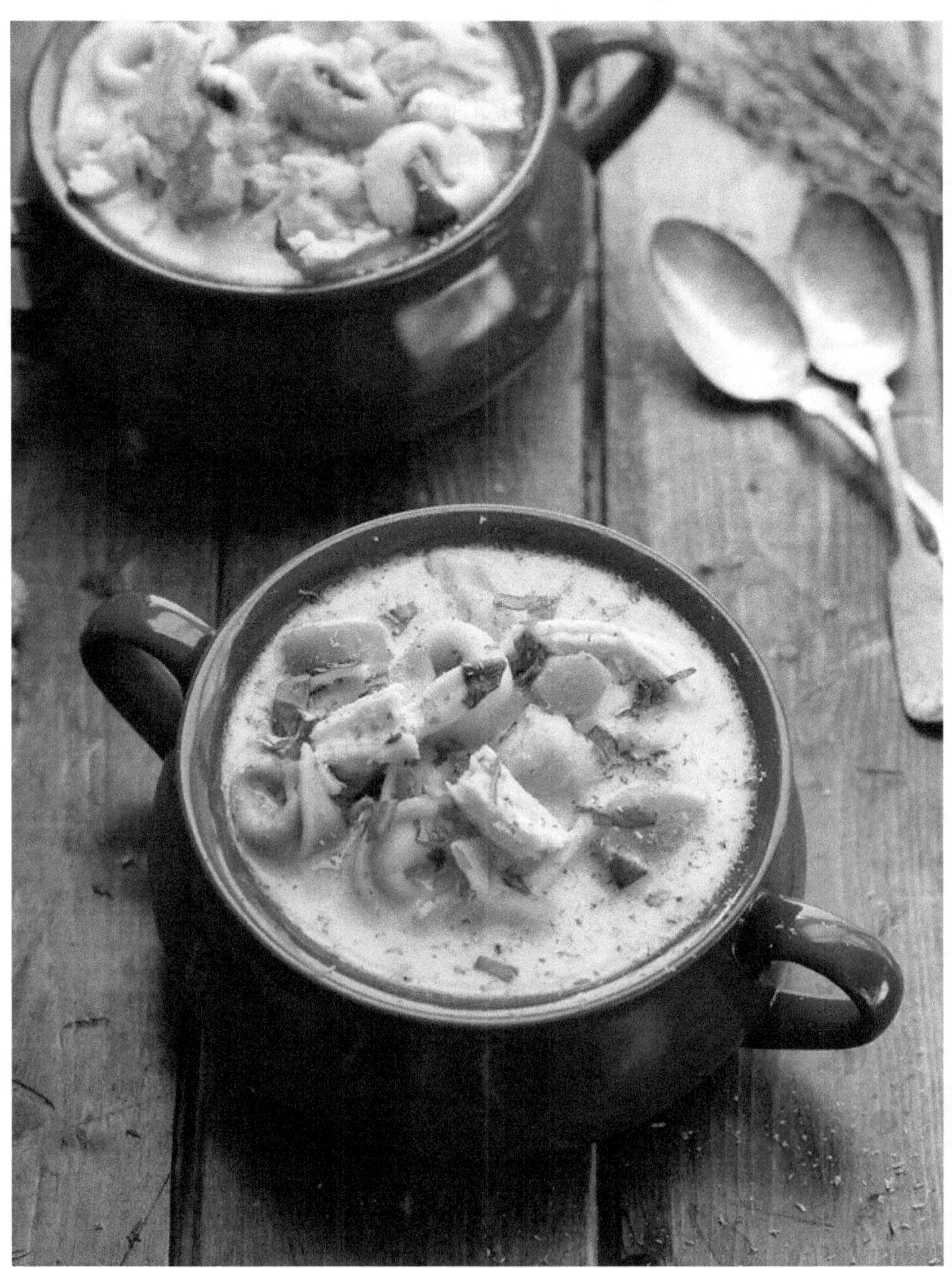